Medical Appointment Book
Belongs To:

_____

If Lost, Please Return To:

_____

_____

_____

Dedication

This Medical Appointment Book is dedicated to all the people who want to keep track of their healthcare appointments, organize your questions, and create a follow-up plan.

You are my inspiration for producing this book and I'm honored to be a part of your record-keeping and ongoing health care.

How to Use this Book

This Medical Appointment Book will help guide you throughout your scheduling, medical concerns, follow up treatments, and more.

Here are examples of tracking and prompts for you to fill in and write the details of your medical appointments:

1. Date - Fill out the information.

2. Appointment Time - Fill out the appointment times.

3. Place of Appointment - Write down the address for the appointment.

4. Medical Appointments/Medical Specialist - Fill out the name of the doctor or specialist.

5. Phone Number - Write phone in this space.

6. Main Concern - Write down your main health concerns.

7. Additional Concerns - Additional space for other areas of concern.

8. Appointment Notes - Jot down any additional information: medications, test results, instructions, etc.

9. Follow-up Tasks - Right down follow up treatments, appointments, etc.

Date: _____ Time: _____

Place of Appointment:

_____

_____

Medical Consultant/Medical Specialist:

_____

Phone Number: _____

Main Concern:

_____
_____
_____

Additional Concerns:

_____
_____

Questions to Ask:

_____
_____
_____

Appointment Notes:

_____
_____
_____
_____
_____

Follow Up Tasks:

_____
_____
_____
_____
_____

Next Appointment:

_____
_____
_____

Date: _____ Time: _____

Place of Appointment:

_____

_____

Medical Consultant/Medical Specialist:

_____

Phone Number: _____

Main Concern:

_____
_____
_____

Additional Concerns:

_____
_____
_____

Questions to Ask:

_____
_____
_____

Appointment Notes:

_____
_____
_____
_____
_____

Follow Up Tasks:

_____
_____
_____
_____
_____

Next Appointment:

_____
_____
_____

Date: _____ Time: _____

Place of Appointment:

_____

_____

Medical Consultant/Medical Specialist:

_____

Phone Number: _____

Main Concern:

_____
_____
_____

Additional Concerns:

_____
_____
_____

Questions to Ask:

_____
_____
_____

Appointment Notes:

_____
_____
_____
_____
_____

Follow Up Tasks:

_____
_____
_____
_____
_____

Next Appointment:

_____
_____
_____

Date: Time:

Place of Appointment:

Medical Consultant/Medical Specialist:

Phone Number:

Main Concern:

_____
_____
_____

Additional Concerns:

_____
_____
_____

Questions to Ask:

_____
_____
_____

Appointment Notes:

_____
_____
_____
_____
_____

Follow Up Tasks:

_____
_____
_____
_____
_____

Next Appointment:

_____
_____
_____

Date: _____ Time: _____

Place of Appointment:

_____

_____

Medical Consultant/Medical Specialist:

_____

Phone Number: _____

Main Concern:

_____
_____
_____

Additional Concerns:

_____
_____
_____

Questions to Ask:

_____
_____
_____

Appointment Notes:

_____
_____
_____
_____
_____

Follow Up Tasks:

_____
_____
_____
_____
_____

Next Appointment:

_____
_____
_____

Date: Time:

Place of Appointment:

Medical Consultant/Medical Specialist:

Phone Number:

Main Concern:

Additional Concerns:

Questions to Ask:

Appointment Notes:

Follow Up Tasks:

Next Appointment:

Date: _____ Time: _____

Place of Appointment:

_____

_____

Medical Consultant/Medical Specialist:

_____

Phone Number: _____

Main Concern:

_____
_____
_____

Additional Concerns:

_____
_____
_____

Questions to Ask:

_____
_____
_____

Appointment Notes:

_____
_____
_____
_____
_____

Follow Up Tasks:

_____
_____
_____
_____
_____

Next Appointment:

_____
_____
_____

Date: _____ Time: _____

Place of Appointment:

_____

_____

Medical Consultant/Medical Specialist:

_____

Phone Number: _____

Main Concern:

_____
_____
_____

Additional Concerns:

_____
_____
_____

Questions to Ask:

_____
_____
_____

Appointment Notes:

_____
_____
_____
_____
_____

Follow Up Tasks:

_____
_____
_____
_____
_____

Next Appointment:

_____
_____
_____

Date: Time:

Place of Appointment:

Medical Consultant/Medical Specialist:

Phone Number:

Main Concern:

_____
_____
_____

Additional Concerns:

_____
_____
_____

Questions to Ask:

_____
_____
_____

Appointment Notes:

_____
_____
_____
_____
_____

Follow Up Tasks:

_____
_____
_____
_____
_____

Next Appointment:

_____
_____
_____

Date: _____ Time: _____

Place of Appointment:

_____

_____

Medical Consultant/Medical Specialist:

_____

Phone Number: _____

Main Concern:

_____
_____
_____

Additional Concerns:

_____
_____
_____

Questions to Ask:

_____
_____
_____

Appointment Notes:

_____
_____
_____
_____
_____

Follow Up Tasks:

_____
_____
_____
_____
_____

Next Appointment:

_____
_____
_____

Date: Time:

Place of Appointment:

Medical Consultant/Medical Specialist:

Phone Number:

Main Concern:

_____
_____
_____

Additional Concerns:

_____
_____
_____

Questions to Ask:

_____
_____
_____

Appointment Notes:

_____
_____
_____
_____
_____

Follow Up Tasks:

_____
_____
_____
_____
_____

Next Appointment:

_____
_____
_____

Date: Time:

Place of Appointment:

Medical Consultant/Medical Specialist:

Phone Number:

Main Concern:

_____
_____
_____

Additional Concerns:

_____
_____
_____

Questions to Ask:

_____
_____
_____

Appointment Notes:

_____
_____
_____
_____
_____

Follow Up Tasks:

_____
_____
_____
_____
_____

Next Appointment:

_____
_____
_____

Date: _____ Time: _____

Place of Appointment:

_____

_____

Medical Consultant/Medical Specialist:

_____

Phone Number: _____

Main Concern:

_____
_____
_____

Additional Concerns:

_____
_____
_____

Questions to Ask:

_____
_____
_____

Appointment Notes:

_____
_____
_____
_____
_____

Follow Up Tasks:

_____
_____
_____
_____
_____

Next Appointment:

_____
_____
_____

Date: _____ Time: _____

Place of Appointment:

_____

_____

Medical Consultant/Medical Specialist:

_____

Phone Number: _____

Main Concern:

_____
_____
_____

Additional Concerns:

_____
_____
_____

Questions to Ask:

_____
_____
_____

Appointment Notes:

_____
_____
_____
_____
_____

Follow Up Tasks:

_____
_____
_____
_____
_____

Next Appointment:

_____
_____
_____

Date: Time:

Place of Appointment:

Medical Consultant/Medical Specialist:

Phone Number:

Main Concern:

_____
_____
_____

Additional Concerns:

_____
_____
_____

Questions to Ask:

_____
_____
_____

Appointment Notes:

_____
_____
_____
_____
_____

Follow Up Tasks:

_____
_____
_____
_____
_____

Next Appointment:

_____
_____
_____

Date: _____ Time: _____

Place of Appointment:

_____

_____

Medical Consultant/Medical Specialist:

_____

Phone Number: _____

Main Concern:

_____
_____
_____

Additional Concerns:

_____
_____
_____

Questions to Ask:

_____
_____
_____

Appointment Notes:

_____
_____
_____
_____
_____

Follow Up Tasks:

_____
_____
_____
_____

Next Appointment:

_____
_____
_____

Date: Time:

Place of Appointment:

Medical Consultant/Medical Specialist:

Phone Number:

Main Concern:

_____
_____
_____

Additional Concerns:

_____
_____
_____

Questions to Ask:

_____
_____
_____

Appointment Notes:

_____
_____
_____
_____
_____

Follow Up Tasks:

_____
_____
_____
_____
_____

Next Appointment:

_____
_____
_____

Date: Time:

Place of Appointment:

Medical Consultant/Medical Specialist:

Phone Number:

Main Concern:

_____
_____
_____

Additional Concerns:

_____
_____
_____

Questions to Ask:

_____
_____
_____

Appointment Notes:

_____
_____
_____
_____
_____

Follow Up Tasks:

_____
_____
_____
_____
_____

Next Appointment:

_____
_____
_____

Date: _____ Time: _____

Place of Appointment:

_____

_____

Medical Consultant/Medical Specialist:

_____

Phone Number: _____

Main Concern:

_____
_____
_____

Additional Concerns:

_____
_____
_____

Questions to Ask:

_____
_____
_____

Appointment Notes:

_____
_____
_____
_____
_____

Follow Up Tasks:

_____
_____
_____
_____
_____

Next Appointment:

_____
_____
_____

Date: Time:

Place of Appointment:

Medical Consultant/Medical Specialist:

Phone Number:

Main Concern:

_____

_____

_____

Additional Concerns:

_____

_____

_____

Questions to Ask:

_____

_____

_____

Appointment Notes:

_____

_____

_____

_____

_____

Follow Up Tasks:

_____

_____

_____

_____

_____

Next Appointment:

_____

_____

_____

Date: Time:

Place of Appointment:

Medical Consultant/Medical Specialist:

Phone Number:

Main Concern:

Additional Concerns:

Questions to Ask:

Appointment Notes:

Follow Up Tasks:

Next Appointment:

Date: Time:

Place of Appointment:

Medical Consultant/Medical Specialist:

Phone Number:

Main Concern:

Additional Concerns:

Questions to Ask:

Appointment Notes:

Follow Up Tasks:

Next Appointment:

Date: _____ Time: _____

Place of Appointment:

_____

_____

Medical Consultant/Medical Specialist:

_____

Phone Number: _____

Main Concern:

_____
_____
_____

Additional Concerns:

_____
_____
_____

Questions to Ask:

_____
_____
_____

Appointment Notes:

_____
_____
_____
_____
_____

Follow Up Tasks:

_____
_____
_____
_____
_____

Next Appointment:

_____
_____
_____

Date: _____ Time: _____

Place of Appointment:

_____

_____

Medical Consultant/Medical Specialist:

_____

Phone Number: _____

Main Concern:

_____
_____
_____

Additional Concerns:

_____
_____
_____

Questions to Ask:

_____
_____
_____

Appointment Notes:

_____
_____
_____
_____
_____

Follow Up Tasks:

_____
_____
_____
_____
_____

Next Appointment:

_____
_____
_____

Date: Time:

Place of Appointment:

Medical Consultant/Medical Specialist:

Phone Number:

Main Concern:

_____
_____
_____

Additional Concerns:

_____
_____
_____

Questions to Ask:

_____
_____
_____

Appointment Notes:

_____
_____
_____
_____
_____

Follow Up Tasks:

_____
_____
_____
_____
_____

Next Appointment:

_____
_____
_____

Date: Time:

Place of Appointment:

Medical Consultant/Medical Specialist:

Phone Number:

Main Concern:

Additional Concerns:

Questions to Ask:

Appointment Notes:

Follow Up Tasks:

Next Appointment:

Date: Time:

Place of Appointment:

Medical Consultant/Medical Specialist:

Phone Number:

Main Concern:

_____
_____
_____

Additional Concerns:

_____
_____
_____

Questions to Ask:

_____
_____
_____

Appointment Notes:

_____
_____
_____
_____
_____

Follow Up Tasks:

_____
_____
_____
_____
_____

Next Appointment:

_____
_____
_____

Date: _____ Time: _____

Place of Appointment:

_____

_____

Medical Consultant/Medical Specialist:

_____

Phone Number: _____

Main Concern:

_____
_____
_____

Additional Concerns:

_____
_____
_____

Questions to Ask:

_____
_____
_____

Appointment Notes:

_____
_____
_____
_____
_____

Follow Up Tasks:

_____
_____
_____
_____
_____

Next Appointment:

_____
_____
_____

Date: _____ Time: _____

Place of Appointment:

_____

_____

Medical Consultant/Medical Specialist:

_____

Phone Number: _____

Main Concern:

_____
_____
_____

Additional Concerns:

_____
_____
_____

Questions to Ask:

_____
_____
_____

Appointment Notes:

_____
_____
_____
_____
_____

Follow Up Tasks:

_____
_____
_____
_____
_____

Next Appointment:

_____
_____
_____

Date: Time:

Place of Appointment:

Medical Consultant/Medical Specialist:

Phone Number:

Main Concern:

_____

_____

_____

Additional Concerns:

_____

_____

_____

Questions to Ask:

_____

_____

_____

Appointment Notes:

_____

_____

_____

_____

_____

Follow Up Tasks:

_____

_____

_____

_____

_____

Next Appointment:

_____

_____

_____

Date: Time:

Place of Appointment:

Medical Consultant/Medical Specialist:

Phone Number:

Main Concern:

_____

_____

_____

Additional Concerns:

_____

_____

Questions to Ask:

_____

_____

Appointment Notes:

_____

_____

_____

_____

Follow Up Tasks:

_____

_____

_____

_____

Next Appointment:

_____

_____

_____

Date: Time:

Place of Appointment:

Medical Consultant/Medical Specialist:

Phone Number:

)

Main Concern:

_____
_____
_____

Additional Concerns:

_____
_____
_____

Questions to Ask:

_____
_____
_____

Appointment Notes:

_____
_____
_____
_____
_____

Follow Up Tasks:

_____
_____
_____
_____
_____

Next Appointment:

_____
_____
_____

Date: Time:

Place of Appointment:

Medical Consultant/Medical Specialist:

Phone Number:

Main Concern:

_____
_____
_____

Additional Concerns:

_____
_____
_____

Questions to Ask:

_____
_____
_____

Appointment Notes:

_____
_____
_____
_____
_____

Follow Up Tasks:

_____
_____
_____
_____
_____

Next Appointment:

_____
_____

Date: _____ Time: _____

Place of Appointment:

_____

_____

Medical Consultant/Medical Specialist:

_____

Phone Number: _____

Main Concern:

_____
_____
_____

Additional Concerns:

_____
_____
_____

Questions to Ask:

_____
_____
_____

Appointment Notes:

_____
_____
_____
_____
_____

Follow Up Tasks:

_____
_____
_____
_____
_____

Next Appointment:

_____
_____
_____

Date: Time:

Place of Appointment:

Medical Consultant/Medical Specialist:

Phone Number:

Main Concern:

_____
_____
_____

Additional Concerns:

_____
_____
_____

Questions to Ask:

_____
_____
_____

Appointment Notes:

_____
_____
_____
_____
_____

Follow Up Tasks:

_____
_____
_____
_____
_____

Next Appointment:

_____
_____
_____

Date: _____ Time: _____

Place of Appointment:

_____

_____

Medical Consultant/Medical Specialist:

_____

Phone Number: _____

Main Concern:

_____
_____
_____

Additional Concerns:

_____
_____
_____

Questions to Ask:

_____
_____
_____

Appointment Notes:

_____
_____
_____
_____
_____

Follow Up Tasks:

_____
_____
_____
_____
_____

Next Appointment:

_____
_____
_____

Date: Time:

Place of Appointment:

Medical Consultant/Medical Specialist:

Phone Number:

Main Concern:

_____
_____
_____

Additional Concerns:

_____
_____
_____

Questions to Ask:

_____
_____
_____

Appointment Notes:

_____
_____
_____
_____
_____

Follow Up Tasks:

_____
_____
_____
_____
_____

Next Appointment:

_____
_____
_____

Date: Time:

Place of Appointment:

Medical Consultant/Medical Specialist:

Phone Number:

Main Concern:

_____
_____
_____

Additional Concerns:

_____
_____
_____

Questions to Ask:

_____
_____
_____

Appointment Notes:

_____
_____
_____
_____
_____

Follow Up Tasks:

_____
_____
_____
_____
_____

Next Appointment:

_____
_____
_____

Date: _____ Time: _____

Place of Appointment:

_____

_____

Medical Consultant/Medical Specialist:

_____

Phone Number: _____

Main Concern:

Additional Concerns:

Questions to Ask:

Appointment Notes:

Follow Up Tasks:

Next Appointment:

Date: Time:

Place of Appointment:

Medical Consultant/Medical Specialist:

Phone Number:

Main Concern:

_____
_____
_____

Additional Concerns:

_____
_____
_____

Questions to Ask:

_____
_____
_____

Appointment Notes:

_____
_____
_____
_____
_____

Follow Up Tasks:

_____
_____
_____
_____
_____

Next Appointment:

_____
_____

Date: _____ Time: _____

Place of Appointment:

_____

_____

Medical Consultant/Medical Specialist:

_____

Phone Number: _____

Main Concern:

_____
_____
_____

Additional Concerns:

_____
_____
_____

Questions to Ask:

_____
_____
_____

Appointment Notes:

_____
_____
_____
_____
_____

Follow Up Tasks:

_____
_____
_____
_____
_____

Next Appointment:

_____
_____
_____

Date: _____ Time: _____

Place of Appointment:
_____

_____

Medical Consultant/Medical Specialist:
_____

Phone Number: _____

Main Concern:
_____
_____
_____

Additional Concerns:
_____
_____
_____

Questions to Ask:
_____
_____
_____

Appointment Notes:
_____
_____
_____
_____
_____

Follow Up Tasks:
_____
_____
_____
_____
_____

Next Appointment:
_____
_____
_____

Date: Time:

Place of Appointment:

Medical Consultant/Medical Specialist:

Phone Number:

Main Concern:

_____
_____
_____

Additional Concerns:

_____
_____
_____

Questions to Ask:

_____
_____
_____

Appointment Notes:

_____
_____
_____
_____
_____

Follow Up Tasks:

_____
_____
_____
_____
_____

Next Appointment:

_____
_____
_____

Date: _____ Time: _____

Place of Appointment:

_____

_____

Medical Consultant/Medical Specialist:

_____

Phone Number: _____

Main Concern:

_____
_____
_____

Additional Concerns:

_____
_____
_____

Questions to Ask:

_____
_____
_____

Appointment Notes:

_____
_____
_____
_____
_____

Follow Up Tasks:

_____
_____
_____
_____
_____

Next Appointment:

_____
_____
_____

Date: Time:

Place of Appointment:

Medical Consultant/Medical Specialist:

Phone Number:

Main Concern:

_____
_____
_____

Additional Concerns:

_____
_____
_____

Questions to Ask:

_____
_____
_____

Appointment Notes:

_____
_____
_____
_____
_____

Follow Up Tasks:

_____
_____
_____
_____
_____

Next Appointment:

_____
_____
_____

Date: _____ Time: _____

Place of Appointment:

_____

_____

Medical Consultant/Medical Specialist:

_____

Phone Number: _____

Main Concern:

_____
_____
_____

Additional Concerns:

_____
_____
_____

Questions to Ask:

_____
_____
_____

Appointment Notes:

_____
_____
_____
_____
_____

Follow Up Tasks:

_____
_____
_____
_____
_____

Next Appointment:

_____
_____
_____

Date: Time:

Place of Appointment:

Medical Consultant/Medical Specialist:

Phone Number:

Main Concern:

_____
_____
_____

Additional Concerns:

_____
_____
_____

Questions to Ask:

_____
_____
_____

Appointment Notes:

_____
_____
_____
_____
_____

Follow Up Tasks:

_____
_____
_____
_____
_____

Next Appointment:

_____
_____
_____

Date: Time:

Place of Appointment:

Medical Consultant/Medical Specialist:

Phone Number:

Main Concern:

_____
_____
_____

Additional Concerns:

_____
_____
_____

Questions to Ask:

_____
_____
_____

Appointment Notes:

_____
_____
_____
_____
_____

Follow Up Tasks:

_____
_____
_____
_____
_____

Next Appointment:

_____
_____
_____

Date: Time:

Place of Appointment:

Medical Consultant/Medical Specialist:

Phone Number:

Main Concern:

_____
_____
_____

Additional Concerns:

_____
_____
_____

Questions to Ask:

_____
_____
_____

Appointment Notes:

_____
_____
_____
_____
_____

Follow Up Tasks:

_____
_____
_____
_____
_____

Next Appointment:

_____
_____
_____

Date: _____ Time: _____

Place of Appointment:

_____

_____

Medical Consultant/Medical Specialist:

_____

Phone Number: _____

Main Concern:

_____
_____
_____

Additional Concerns:

_____
_____
_____

Questions to Ask:

_____
_____
_____

Appointment Notes:

_____
_____
_____
_____
_____

Follow Up Tasks:

_____
_____
_____
_____
_____

Next Appointment:

_____
_____
_____

Date: _____ Time: _____

Place of Appointment: _____

_____

Medical Consultant/Medical Specialist: _____

Phone Number: _____

Main Concern:

_____
_____
_____

Additional Concerns:

_____
_____
_____

Questions to Ask:

_____
_____
_____

Appointment Notes:

_____
_____
_____
_____
_____

Follow Up Tasks:

_____
_____
_____
_____
_____

Next Appointment:

_____
_____
_____

Date: _____ Time: _____

Place of Appointment:

_____

_____

Medical Consultant/Medical Specialist:

_____

Phone Number: _____

Main Concern:

_____
_____
_____

Additional Concerns:

_____
_____
_____

Questions to Ask:

_____
_____
_____

Appointment Notes:

_____
_____
_____
_____
_____

Follow Up Tasks:

_____
_____
_____
_____
_____

Next Appointment:

_____
_____
_____

Date: _____ Time: _____

Place of Appointment:

_____

_____

Medical Consultant/Medical Specialist:

_____

Phone Number: _____

Main Concern:

_____
_____
_____

Additional Concerns:

_____
_____
_____

Questions to Ask:

_____
_____
_____

Appointment Notes:

_____
_____
_____
_____
_____

Follow Up Tasks:

_____
_____
_____
_____
_____

Next Appointment:

_____
_____
_____

Date: Time:

Place of Appointment:

Medical Consultant/Medical Specialist:

Phone Number:

Main Concern:

_____
_____
_____

Additional Concerns:

_____
_____
_____

Questions to Ask:

_____
_____
_____

Appointment Notes:

_____
_____
_____
_____
_____

Follow Up Tasks:

_____
_____
_____
_____
_____

Next Appointment:

_____
_____
_____

Date: _____ Time: _____

Place of Appointment:

_____

_____

Medical Consultant/Medical Specialist:

_____

Phone Number: _____

Main Concern:

_____
_____
_____

Additional Concerns:

_____
_____
_____

Questions to Ask:

_____
_____
_____

Appointment Notes:

_____
_____
_____
_____
_____

Follow Up Tasks:

_____
_____
_____
_____
_____

Next Appointment:

_____
_____
_____

Date: Time:

Place of Appointment:

Medical Consultant/Medical Specialist:

Phone Number:

Main Concern:

_____
_____
_____

Additional Concerns:

_____
_____
_____

Questions to Ask:

_____
_____
_____

Appointment Notes:

_____
_____
_____
_____
_____

Follow Up Tasks:

_____
_____
_____
_____

Next Appointment:

_____
_____
_____

Date: _____ Time: _____

Place of Appointment:

_____

_____

Medical Consultant/Medical Specialist:

_____

Phone Number: _____

Main Concern:

_____
_____
_____

Additional Concerns:

_____
_____
_____

Questions to Ask:

_____
_____
_____

Appointment Notes:

_____
_____
_____
_____
_____

Follow Up Tasks:

_____
_____
_____
_____
_____

Next Appointment:

_____
_____
_____

Date: _____ Time: _____

Place of Appointment:

_____

_____

Medical Consultant/Medical Specialist:

_____

Phone Number: _____

Main Concern:

_____
_____
_____

Additional Concerns:

_____
_____
_____

Questions to Ask:

_____
_____
_____

Appointment Notes:

_____
_____
_____
_____
_____

Follow Up Tasks:

_____
_____
_____
_____
_____

Next Appointment:

_____
_____
_____

Date: _____ Time: _____

Place of Appointment:

_____

_____

Medical Consultant/Medical Specialist:

_____

Phone Number: _____

Main Concern:

_____
_____
_____

Additional Concerns:

_____
_____
_____

Questions to Ask:

_____
_____
_____

Appointment Notes:

_____
_____
_____
_____
_____

Follow Up Tasks:

_____
_____
_____
_____
_____

Next Appointment:

_____
_____
_____

Date: Time:

Place of Appointment:

Medical Consultant/Medical Specialist:

Phone Number:

Main Concern:

_____
_____
_____

Additional Concerns:

_____
_____
_____

Questions to Ask:

_____
_____
_____

Appointment Notes:

_____
_____
_____
_____
_____

Follow Up Tasks:

_____
_____
_____
_____
_____

Next Appointment:

_____
_____
_____

Date: Time:

Place of Appointment:

Medical Consultant/Medical Specialist:

Phone Number:

Main Concern:

_____
_____
_____

Additional Concerns:

_____
_____
_____

Questions to Ask:

_____
_____
_____

Appointment Notes:

_____
_____
_____
_____
_____

Follow Up Tasks:

_____
_____
_____
_____
_____

Next Appointment:

_____
_____
_____

Date: _____ Time: _____

Place of Appointment:

_____

_____

Medical Consultant/Medical Specialist:

_____

Phone Number: _____

Main Concern:

_____
_____
_____

Additional Concerns:

_____
_____
_____

Questions to Ask:

_____
_____
_____

Appointment Notes:

_____
_____
_____
_____
_____

Follow Up Tasks:

_____
_____
_____
_____
_____

Next Appointment:

_____
_____
_____

Date: .... Time: ....

Place of Appointment:

....

....

Medical Consultant/Medical Specialist:

....

Phone Number: ....

Main Concern:

_____
_____
_____

Additional Concerns:

_____
_____
_____

Questions to Ask:

_____
_____
_____

Appointment Notes:

_____
_____
_____
_____
_____

Follow Up Tasks:

_____
_____
_____
_____
_____

Next Appointment:

_____
_____
_____

Date: _____ Time: _____

Place of Appointment:

_____

_____

Medical Consultant/Medical Specialist:

_____

Phone Number: _____

Main Concern:

_____
_____
_____

Additional Concerns:

_____
_____
_____

Questions to Ask:

_____
_____
_____

Appointment Notes:

_____
_____
_____
_____
_____

Follow Up Tasks:

_____
_____
_____
_____

Next Appointment:

_____
_____
_____

Date: Time:

Place of Appointment:

Medical Consultant/Medical Specialist:

Phone Number:

Main Concern:

_____
_____
_____

Additional Concerns:

_____
_____
_____

Questions to Ask:

_____
_____
_____

Appointment Notes:

_____
_____
_____
_____
_____

Follow Up Tasks:

_____
_____
_____
_____
_____

Next Appointment:

_____
_____
_____

Date: _____ Time: _____

Place of Appointment:

_____

_____

Medical Consultant/Medical Specialist:

_____

Phone Number: _____

Main Concern:

_____
_____
_____

Additional Concerns:

_____
_____
_____

Questions to Ask:

_____
_____
_____

Appointment Notes:

_____
_____
_____
_____
_____

Follow Up Tasks:

_____
_____
_____
_____

Next Appointment:

_____
_____
_____

Date: Time:

Place of Appointment:

Medical Consultant/Medical Specialist:

Phone Number:

Main Concern:

_____
_____
_____

Additional Concerns:

_____
_____
_____

Questions to Ask:

_____
_____
_____

Appointment Notes:

_____
_____
_____
_____
_____

Follow Up Tasks:

_____
_____
_____
_____
_____

Next Appointment:

_____
_____
_____

Date: Time:

Place of Appointment:

Medical Consultant/Medical Specialist:

Phone Number:

Main Concern:

_____
_____
_____

Additional Concerns:

_____
_____
_____

Questions to Ask:

_____
_____
_____

Appointment Notes:

_____
_____
_____
_____
_____

Follow Up Tasks:

_____
_____
_____
_____
_____

Next Appointment:

_____
_____
_____

Date: _____ Time: _____

Place of Appointment:

_____

_____

Medical Consultant/Medical Specialist:

_____

Phone Number: _____

Main Concern:

_____
_____
_____

Additional Concerns:

_____
_____
_____

Questions to Ask:

_____
_____
_____

Appointment Notes:

_____
_____
_____
_____
_____

Follow Up Tasks:

_____
_____
_____
_____
_____

Next Appointment:

_____
_____
_____

Date: _____ Time: _____

Place of Appointment:

_____

_____

Medical Consultant/Medical Specialist:

_____

Phone Number: _____

Main Concern:

_____
_____
_____

Additional Concerns:

_____
_____
_____

Questions to Ask:

_____
_____
_____

Appointment Notes:

_____
_____
_____
_____
_____

Follow Up Tasks:

_____
_____
_____
_____
_____

Next Appointment:

_____
_____
_____

Date: Time:

Place of Appointment:

Medical Consultant/Medical Specialist:

Phone Number:

Main Concern:

_____
_____
_____

Additional Concerns:

_____
_____
_____

Questions to Ask:

_____
_____
_____

Appointment Notes:

_____
_____
_____
_____
_____

Follow Up Tasks:

_____
_____
_____
_____
_____

Next Appointment:

_____
_____
_____

Date: _____ Time: _____

Place of Appointment:

_____

_____

Medical Consultant/Medical Specialist:

_____

Phone Number: _____

Main Concern:

_____
_____
_____

Additional Concerns:

_____
_____
_____

Questions to Ask:

_____
_____
_____

Appointment Notes:

_____
_____
_____
_____
_____

Follow Up Tasks:

_____
_____
_____
_____
_____

Next Appointment:

_____
_____
_____

Date: _____ Time: _____

Place of Appointment:

_____

_____

Medical Consultant/Medical Specialist:

_____

Phone Number: _____

Main Concern:

_____
_____
_____

Additional Concerns:

_____
_____
_____

Questions to Ask:

_____
_____
_____

Appointment Notes:

_____
_____
_____
_____
_____

Follow Up Tasks:

_____
_____
_____
_____
_____

Next Appointment:

_____
_____
_____

Date: _____ Time: _____

Place of Appointment:

_____

_____

Medical Consultant/Medical Specialist:

_____

Phone Number: _____

Main Concern:

_____
_____
_____

Additional Concerns:

_____
_____
_____

Questions to Ask:

_____
_____
_____

Appointment Notes:

_____
_____
_____
_____
_____

Follow Up Tasks:

_____
_____
_____
_____
_____

Next Appointment:

_____
_____
_____

Date: Time:

Place of Appointment:

Medical Consultant/Medical Specialist:

Phone Number:

Main Concern:

_____
_____
_____

Additional Concerns:

_____
_____
_____

Questions to Ask:

_____
_____
_____

Appointment Notes:

_____
_____
_____
_____
_____

Follow Up Tasks:

_____
_____
_____
_____
_____

Next Appointment:

_____
_____
_____

Date: _____ Time: _____

Place of Appointment:

_____

_____

Medical Consultant/Medical Specialist:

_____

Phone Number: _____

Main Concern:

_____
_____
_____

Additional Concerns:

_____
_____
_____

Questions to Ask:

_____
_____
_____

Appointment Notes:

_____
_____
_____
_____
_____

Follow Up Tasks:

_____
_____
_____
_____
_____

Next Appointment:

_____
_____
_____

Date: _____ Time: _____

Place of Appointment:

_____

_____

Medical Consultant/Medical Specialist:

_____

Phone Number: _____

Main Concern:

_____
_____
_____

Additional Concerns:

_____
_____
_____

Questions to Ask:

_____
_____
_____

Appointment Notes:

_____
_____
_____
_____
_____

Follow Up Tasks:

_____
_____
_____
_____
_____

Next Appointment:

_____
_____
_____

Date: _____ Time: _____
Place of Appointment:
_____

_____

Medical Consultant/Medical Specialist:
_____

Phone Number: _____

Main Concern:
_____
_____
_____

Additional Concerns:
_____
_____
_____

Questions to Ask:
_____
_____
_____

Appointment Notes:
_____
_____
_____
_____
_____

Follow Up Tasks:
_____
_____
_____
_____

Next Appointment:
_____
_____
_____

Date: Time:

Place of Appointment:

Medical Consultant/Medical Specialist:

Phone Number:

Main Concern:

_____
_____
_____

Additional Concerns:

_____
_____
_____

Questions to Ask:

_____
_____
_____

Appointment Notes:

_____
_____
_____
_____
_____
_____

Follow Up Tasks:

_____
_____
_____
_____
_____
_____

Next Appointment:

_____
_____
_____

Date: _____ Time: _____

Place of Appointment:

_____

_____

Medical Consultant/Medical Specialist:

_____

Phone Number: _____

Main Concern:

_____
_____
_____

Additional Concerns:

_____
_____
_____

Questions to Ask:

_____
_____
_____

Appointment Notes:

_____
_____
_____
_____
_____

Follow Up Tasks:

_____
_____
_____
_____
_____

Next Appointment:

_____
_____
_____

Date: _____ Time: _____

Place of Appointment:

_____

_____

Medical Consultant/Medical Specialist:

_____

Phone Number: _____

Main Concern:

_____
_____
_____

Additional Concerns:

_____
_____
_____

Questions to Ask:

_____
_____
_____

Appointment Notes:

_____
_____
_____
_____
_____

Follow Up Tasks:

_____
_____
_____
_____
_____

Next Appointment:

_____
_____
_____

Date: Time:

Place of Appointment:

Medical Consultant/Medical Specialist:

Phone Number:

Main Concern:

_____
_____
_____

Additional Concerns:

_____
_____
_____

Questions to Ask:

_____
_____
_____

Appointment Notes:

_____
_____
_____
_____
_____

Follow Up Tasks:

_____
_____
_____
_____
_____

Next Appointment:

_____
_____
_____

Date: _____ Time: _____

Place of Appointment:

_____

_____

Medical Consultant/Medical Specialist:

_____

Phone Number: _____

Main Concern:

_____
_____
_____

Additional Concerns:

_____
_____
_____

Questions to Ask:

_____
_____
_____

Appointment Notes:

_____
_____
_____
_____
_____

Follow Up Tasks:

_____
_____
_____
_____
_____

Next Appointment:

_____
_____
_____

Date: Time:

Place of Appointment:

Medical Consultant/Medical Specialist:

Phone Number:

Main Concern:

_____
_____
_____

Additional Concerns:

_____
_____
_____

Questions to Ask:

_____
_____
_____

Appointment Notes:

_____
_____
_____
_____
_____

Follow Up Tasks:

_____
_____
_____
_____
_____

Next Appointment:

_____
_____
_____

Date: _____ Time: _____

Place of Appointment:

_____

_____

Medical Consultant/Medical Specialist:

_____

Phone Number: _____

Main Concern:

_____
_____
_____

Additional Concerns:

_____
_____
_____

Questions to Ask:

_____
_____
_____

Appointment Notes:

_____
_____
_____
_____
_____

Follow Up Tasks:

_____
_____
_____
_____
_____

Next Appointment:

_____
_____
_____

Date: Time:

Place of Appointment:

Medical Consultant/Medical Specialist:

Phone Number:

Main Concern:

_____
_____
_____

Additional Concerns:

_____
_____
_____

Questions to Ask:

_____
_____
_____

Appointment Notes:

_____
_____
_____
_____
_____

Follow Up Tasks:

_____
_____
_____
_____
_____

Next Appointment:

_____
_____
_____

Date: Time:

Place of Appointment:

Medical Consultant/Medical Specialist:

Phone Number:

Main Concern:

_____
_____
_____

Additional Concerns:

_____
_____
_____

Questions to Ask:

_____
_____
_____

Appointment Notes:

_____
_____
_____
_____
_____

Follow Up Tasks:

_____
_____
_____
_____
_____

Next Appointment:

_____
_____
_____

Date: _____ Time: _____

Place of Appointment:

_____

_____

Medical Consultant/Medical Specialist:

_____

Phone Number: _____

Main Concern:

_____
_____
_____

Additional Concerns:

_____
_____
_____

Questions to Ask:

_____
_____
_____

Appointment Notes:

_____
_____
_____
_____
_____

Follow Up Tasks:

_____
_____
_____
_____
_____

Next Appointment:

_____
_____

Date: _____ Time: _____

Place of Appointment:

_____

_____

Medical Consultant/Medical Specialist:

_____

Phone Number: _____

Main Concern:

_____
_____
_____

Additional Concerns:

_____
_____
_____

Questions to Ask:

_____
_____
_____

Appointment Notes:

_____
_____
_____
_____
_____

Follow Up Tasks:

_____
_____
_____
_____
_____

Next Appointment:

_____
_____
_____

Date: Time:

Place of Appointment:

Medical Consultant/Medical Specialist:

Phone Number:

Main Concern:

_____

_____

_____

Additional Concerns:

_____

_____

_____

Questions to Ask:

_____

_____

_____

Appointment Notes:

_____

_____

_____

_____

_____

Follow Up Tasks:

_____

_____

_____

_____

_____

Next Appointment:

_____

_____

_____

Date: Time:

Place of Appointment:

Medical Consultant/Medical Specialist:

Phone Number:

Main Concern:

_____
_____
_____

Additional Concerns:

_____
_____

Questions to Ask:

_____
_____
_____

Appointment Notes:

_____
_____
_____
_____
_____

Follow Up Tasks:

_____
_____
_____
_____
_____

Next Appointment:

_____
_____
_____

Date: Time:

Place of Appointment:

Medical Consultant/Medical Specialist:

Phone Number:

Main Concern:

_____
_____
_____

Additional Concerns:

_____
_____
_____

Questions to Ask:

_____
_____
_____

Appointment Notes:

_____
_____
_____
_____
_____

Follow Up Tasks:

_____
_____
_____
_____
_____

Next Appointment:

_____
_____
_____

Date: Time:

Place of Appointment:

Medical Consultant/Medical Specialist:

Phone Number:

Main Concern:

_____

_____

_____

Additional Concerns:

_____

_____

_____

Questions to Ask:

_____

_____

_____

Appointment Notes:

_____

_____

_____

_____

_____

Follow Up Tasks:

_____

_____

_____

_____

_____

Next Appointment:

_____

_____

_____

Date: Time:

Place of Appointment:

Medical Consultant/Medical Specialist:

Phone Number:

Main Concern:

_____
_____
_____

Additional Concerns:

_____
_____
_____

Questions to Ask:

_____
_____
_____

Appointment Notes:

_____
_____
_____
_____
_____

Follow Up Tasks:

_____
_____
_____
_____
_____

Next Appointment:

_____
_____

Date: _____ Time: _____

Place of Appointment:

_____

_____

Medical Consultant/Medical Specialist:

_____

Phone Number: _____

Main Concern:

_____
_____
_____

Additional Concerns:

_____
_____
_____

Questions to Ask:

_____
_____
_____

Appointment Notes:

_____
_____
_____
_____
_____
_____

Follow Up Tasks:

_____
_____
_____
_____

Next Appointment:

_____
_____
_____

Date: Time:

Place of Appointment:

Medical Consultant/Medical Specialist:

Phone Number:

Main Concern:

_____

_____

_____

Additional Concerns:

_____

_____

_____

Questions to Ask:

_____

_____

_____

Appointment Notes:

_____

_____

_____

_____

_____

Follow Up Tasks:

_____

_____

_____

_____

_____

Next Appointment:

_____

_____

_____

Date: _____ Time: _____

Place of Appointment:

_____

_____

Medical Consultant/Medical Specialist:

_____

Phone Number: _____

Main Concern:

_____
_____
_____

Additional Concerns:

_____
_____

Questions to Ask:

_____
_____
_____

Appointment Notes:

_____
_____
_____
_____
_____

Follow Up Tasks:

_____
_____
_____
_____
_____

Next Appointment:

_____
_____
_____

Date: _____ Time: _____

Place of Appointment:

_____

_____

Medical Consultant/Medical Specialist:

_____

Phone Number: _____

Main Concern:

_____

_____

_____

Additional Concerns:

_____

_____

_____

Questions to Ask:

_____

_____

_____

Appointment Notes:

_____

_____

_____

_____

_____

Follow Up Tasks:

_____

_____

_____

_____

_____

Next Appointment:

_____

_____

_____

Date: _____ Time: _____

Place of Appointment:

_____

_____

Medical Consultant/Medical Specialist:

_____

Phone Number: _____

Main Concern:

_____
_____
_____

Additional Concerns:

_____
_____
_____

Questions to Ask:

_____
_____
_____

Appointment Notes:

_____
_____
_____
_____
_____

Follow Up Tasks:

_____
_____
_____
_____
_____

Next Appointment:

_____
_____
_____

Date: _____ Time: _____
Place of Appointment:

_____

_____

Medical Consultant/Medical Specialist:

_____

Phone Number: _____

Main Concern:

_____
_____
_____

Additional Concerns:

_____
_____
_____

Questions to Ask:

_____
_____
_____

Appointment Notes:

_____
_____
_____
_____
_____

Follow Up Tasks:

_____
_____
_____
_____
_____

Next Appointment:

_____
_____
_____

Date: _____ Time: _____

Place of Appointment:

_____

_____

Medical Consultant/Medical Specialist:

_____

Phone Number: _____

Main Concern:

_____
_____
_____

Additional Concerns:

_____
_____
_____

Questions to Ask:

_____
_____
_____

Appointment Notes:

_____
_____
_____
_____
_____

Follow Up Tasks:

_____
_____
_____
_____

Next Appointment:

_____
_____
_____

Date: Time:

Place of Appointment:

Medical Consultant/Medical Specialist:

Phone Number:

Main Concern:

_____
_____
_____

Additional Concerns:

_____
_____
_____

Questions to Ask:

_____
_____
_____

Appointment Notes:

_____
_____
_____
_____
_____

Follow Up Tasks:

_____
_____
_____
_____
_____

Next Appointment:

_____
_____
_____

Date: _____ Time: _____

Place of Appointment:

_____

_____

Medical Consultant/Medical Specialist:

_____

Phone Number: _____

Main Concern:

_____
_____
_____

Additional Concerns:

_____
_____
_____

Questions to Ask:

_____
_____
_____

Appointment Notes:

_____
_____
_____
_____
_____

Follow Up Tasks:

_____
_____
_____
_____
_____

Next Appointment:

_____
_____
_____

Date: Time:

Place of Appointment:

Medical Consultant/Medical Specialist:

Phone Number:

Main Concern:

Additional Concerns:

Questions to Ask:

Appointment Notes:

Follow Up Tasks:

Next Appointment:

Date: Time:

Place of Appointment:

Medical Consultant/Medical Specialist:

Phone Number:

Main Concern:

_____
_____
_____

Additional Concerns:

_____
_____
_____

Questions to Ask:

_____
_____
_____

Appointment Notes:

_____
_____
_____
_____
_____

Follow Up Tasks:

_____
_____
_____
_____
_____

Next Appointment:

_____
_____
_____

Date: _____ Time: _____

Place of Appointment:

_____

_____

Medical Consultant/Medical Specialist:

_____

Phone Number: _____

Main Concern:

_____
_____
_____

Additional Concerns:

_____
_____
_____

Questions to Ask:

_____
_____
_____

Appointment Notes:

_____
_____
_____
_____
_____

Follow Up Tasks:

_____
_____
_____
_____
_____

Next Appointment:

_____
_____
_____

Date: _____ Time: _____

Place of Appointment:

_____

_____

Medical Consultant/Medical Specialist:

_____

Phone Number: _____

Main Concern:

_____
_____
_____

Additional Concerns:

_____
_____
_____

Questions to Ask:

_____
_____
_____

Appointment Notes:

_____
_____
_____
_____
_____

Follow Up Tasks:

_____
_____
_____
_____
_____

Next Appointment:

_____
_____
_____

Date: _____ Time: _____

Place of Appointment:

_____

_____

Medical Consultant/Medical Specialist:

_____

Phone Number: _____

Main Concern:

_____
_____
_____

Additional Concerns:

_____
_____
_____

Questions to Ask:

_____
_____
_____

Appointment Notes:

_____
_____
_____
_____
_____

Follow Up Tasks:

_____
_____
_____
_____
_____

Next Appointment:

_____
_____
_____

Date: Time:

Place of Appointment:

Medical Consultant/Medical Specialist:

Phone Number:

Main Concern:

_____
_____
_____

Additional Concerns:

_____
_____
_____

Questions to Ask:

_____
_____
_____

Appointment Notes:

_____
_____
_____
_____
_____
_____

Follow Up Tasks:

_____
_____
_____
_____
_____
_____

Next Appointment:

_____
_____
_____

Date: Time:

Place of Appointment:

Medical Consultant/Medical Specialist:

Phone Number:

Main Concern:

_____

_____

_____

Additional Concerns:

_____

_____

_____

Questions to Ask:

_____

_____

_____

Appointment Notes:

_____

_____

_____

_____

_____

Follow Up Tasks:

_____

_____

_____

_____

_____

Next Appointment:

_____

_____

_____

Date: _____ Time: _____

Place of Appointment:

_____

_____

Medical Consultant/Medical Specialist:

_____

Phone Number: _____

Main Concern:

_____
_____
_____

Additional Concerns:

_____
_____
_____

Questions to Ask:

_____
_____
_____

Appointment Notes:

_____
_____
_____
_____
_____

Follow Up Tasks:

_____
_____
_____
_____
_____

Next Appointment:

_____
_____
_____

Date: _____ Time: _____

Place of Appointment:

_____

_____

Medical Consultant/Medical Specialist:

_____

Phone Number: _____

Main Concern:

_____
_____
_____

Additional Concerns:

_____
_____
_____

Questions to Ask:

_____
_____
_____

Appointment Notes:

_____
_____
_____
_____
_____

Follow Up Tasks:

_____
_____
_____
_____
_____

Next Appointment:

_____
_____
_____

Date: _____ Time: _____

Place of Appointment:

_____

_____

Medical Consultant/Medical Specialist:

_____

Phone Number: _____

Main Concern:

_____
_____
_____

Additional Concerns:

_____
_____
_____

Questions to Ask:

_____
_____
_____

Appointment Notes:

_____
_____
_____
_____
_____

Follow Up Tasks:

_____
_____
_____
_____
_____

Next Appointment:

_____
_____
_____

Date: Time:

Place of Appointment:

Medical Consultant/Medical Specialist:

Phone Number:

Main Concern:

_____
_____
_____

Additional Concerns:

_____
_____
_____

Questions to Ask:

_____
_____
_____

Appointment Notes:

_____
_____
_____
_____
_____

Follow Up Tasks:

_____
_____
_____
_____
_____

Next Appointment:

_____
_____
_____

Date: Time:
Place of Appointment:

Medical Consultant/Medical Specialist:

Phone Number:

Main Concern:

_____
_____
_____

Additional Concerns:

_____
_____
_____

Questions to Ask:

_____
_____
_____

Appointment Notes:

_____
_____
_____
_____
_____

Follow Up Tasks:

_____
_____
_____
_____
_____

Next Appointment:

_____
_____
_____

Date: Time:

Place of Appointment:

Medical Consultant/Medical Specialist:

Phone Number:

Main Concern:

Additional Concerns:

Questions to Ask:

Appointment Notes:

Follow Up Tasks:

Next Appointment:

Date: Time:

Place of Appointment:

Medical Consultant/Medical Specialist:

Phone Number:

Main Concern:

_____
_____
_____

Additional Concerns:

_____
_____
_____

Questions to Ask:

_____
_____
_____

Appointment Notes:

_____
_____
_____
_____
_____

Follow Up Tasks:

_____
_____
_____
_____
_____

Next Appointment:

_____
_____
_____

Date: Time:

Place of Appointment:

Medical Consultant/Medical Specialist:

Phone Number:

Main Concern:

_____
_____
_____

Additional Concerns:

_____
_____
_____

Questions to Ask:

_____
_____
_____

Appointment Notes:

_____
_____
_____
_____
_____

Follow Up Tasks:

_____
_____
_____
_____
_____

Next Appointment:

_____
_____
_____

Date: Time:

Place of Appointment:

Medical Consultant/Medical Specialist:

Phone Number:

Main Concern:

Additional Concerns:

Questions to Ask:

Appointment Notes:

Follow Up Tasks:

Next Appointment:

Date: Time:

Place of Appointment:

Medical Consultant/Medical Specialist:

Phone Number:

Main Concern:

_____

_____

_____

Additional Concerns:

_____

_____

_____

Questions to Ask:

_____

_____

_____

Appointment Notes:

_____

_____

_____

_____

_____

Follow Up Tasks:

_____

_____

_____

_____

_____

Next Appointment:

_____

_____

_____